YOUR KNOWLEDGE HAS VALUE

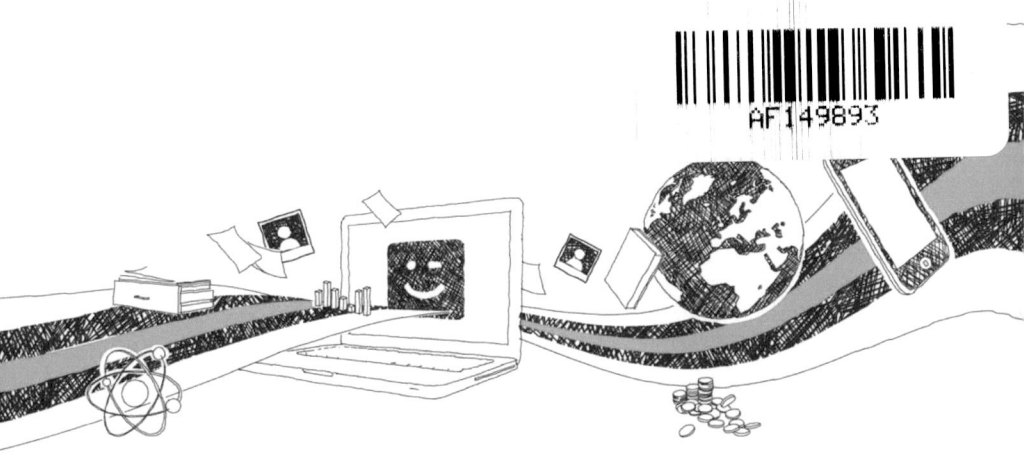

- We will publish your bachelor's and
  master's thesis, essays and papers

- Your own eBook and book -
  sold worldwide in all relevant shops

- Earn money with each sale

Upload your text at www.GRIN.com
and publish for free

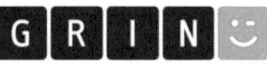

Ellen Garcia

Breast feeding for cognitive development

GRIN Publishing

Bibliographic information published by the German National Library:

The German National Library lists this publication in the National Bibliography;
detailed bibliographic data are available on the Internet at http://dnb.dnb.de .

This book is copyright material and must not be copied, reproduced, transferred,
distributed, leased, licensed or publicly performed or used in any way except as
specifically permitted in writing by the publishers, as allowed under the terms and
conditions under which it was purchased or as strictly permitted by applicable
copyright law. Any unauthorized distribution or use of this text may be a direct
infringement of the author s and publisher s rights and those responsible may be
liable in law accordingly.

Imprint:

Copyright © 2012 GRIN Verlag GmbH
Print and binding: Books on Demand GmbH, Norderstedt Germany
ISBN: 978-3-656-63316-7

This book at GRIN:

http://www.grin.com/en/e-book/271552/breast-feeding-for-cognitive-development

GRIN - Your knowledge has value

Since its foundation in 1998, GRIN has specialized in publishing academic texts by students, college teachers and other academics as e-book and printed book. The website www.grin.com is an ideal platform for presenting term papers, final papers, scientific essays, dissertations and specialist books.

Visit us on the internet:

http://www.grin.com/

http://www.facebook.com/grincom

http://www.twitter.com/grin_com

The Importance of Breast feeding for Cognitive Development

As usual, traditions that have been followed for long always form subjects of debate. Traditionally women used to breast feed their infants till the next child is born or at least for a year without any complain. The situation has however changed as mothers now opt for infant formula readily available in our markets. This has raised a serious issue of debate as nutritionists and pediatrics as a whole still recommend six months exclusive breast feeding while manufactures of these products are capitalizing on the fact that today's mothers are more busy thus has little time for their babies. Breast feeding had traditionally been associated with the development of strong immune system for babies, the single most reason why pediatrics always recommend six months exclusive breast feeding period to mothers. Studies currently have tried to address other reasons why breast feeding should be treated with importance. One of this reasons that has received renowned attention is the connection between breastfeeding and cognitive development. The importance of breast feeding for cognitive development was first explored by Hoefer and Hardy (1929) when they carried out a study on *"later development of breast fed and artificially fed infants."* Since then this topic has been researched by many scholars. While most scholars argue that breast fed children ranks high on clinical studies done on cognitive function, others argue that these perceived differences can be attributed to other factors such as maternal education or socio-economic factors (Anderson, 1999). The development of cognitive functions in infants is of course a more complex process being influenced by many factors including genetics as well as environmental factors. The role played by nutrition an in this case breastfeeding cannot be under estimated either. This piece of work therefore seeks to address the role played by breast feeding in cognitive development. This is achieved through review of available literature including previous research on this topic. Recommendations on best practices as well as proposal for future research are also provided.

Review of literature

Breast fed children score good grades than those formula fed children? Is this some sort of a campaign slogan by supporters of breast feeding? Are there facts to support this luring statement? One of the important stories that our writers have not given coverage is perhaps the demonstrated direct relationship between breast milk and brain development. Considering the fact that at birth the brain is probably one third formed and the rest of the development takes place during the first few years after birth thus need for intake of nutrients that contribute directly. Studies have demonstrated that while cow milk would be best for the development of strong bones, breast milk is very essential for cognitive development. One of the most researched and a reported benefit of breastfeeding is its links with high IQ and measurable outputs in cognitive development as compared with artificial feeds (Anderson, 1999). The topic of breastfeeding and its role on cognitive development is not a new topic in the world of clinical research. This topic has been studied by many for over decades. While a general agreement exist among scholars that breast feeding is associated with high intellectual capacity, it is however unclear whether this advantage should solely be attributed to breastfeeding or other interacting factors.

Studies carried out by various scholars have revealed that children who were breastfed perform better than their counterparts in tests of cognition, intellectual and verbal. These results have been similar regardless of whether the child was born at term or preterm. However confusions have always arose based on two sources: the intimacy between the mother and baby derived from breast feeding may be very significant in the development; and there is a very big difference in terms of education and socio-economic status between mothers who choose to breast feed and those who opt not to, thus maternal characteristics are equally very important (Lucas 1992). Given these confounding factors, many studies have tried to adjust their methodology to incorporate them but the results still accord breast feeding a remarkable importance in influencing cognitive development in children.

A study carried by Adair and Daniels (2005) in which case the intimacy was eliminated by feeding infants through nasogastric tube as opposed to direct sucking revealed very pleasing results. Even after eliminating intimacy, there was clear evidence that children who were continually fed on breast milk had a developmental advantage both in Bayley Mental Development Index at 18 months and IQ at 7.5-8 years for those born post term. A comparison study carried out on children whose mothers continue to breast feed directly reveals similar results showing that regardless of intimacy, breast feeding plays a significant role in cognitive development.

Hoefer and Hardy (1929) in trying to establish the importance of breastfeeding for cognitive development in the US during the years 1915-1921 revealed that children who were breast fed did better than those artificially fed. He however discovered that exclusive breast

2

feeding after 9 months can be very harmful to the development as children under this category performed less well.

One of the most significant studies in this field was carried out by Anderson (1999) in their meta-analysis studies. They recorded a consistent IQ differences in the range of 2-5 points favoring children who were breast fed over those who survived on the formula. Most of the meta-analysis studies were conducted on subjects who were born at term so some argue that their results may not hold water for those born pre-term. Lucas (1992) carried out a similar randomized study using subjects who were born pre-term and came up with similar results although with a much larger difference of 8 points.

Adair and Melissa (2005) studied the relationship between breastfeeding and cognitive development in Filipino children. To broaden their study they came up with a broader approach whereby they inversely correlated breast feeding with other factors such as healthy maternal behaviors and socioeconomic advantages. The study was followed from the period of birth to middle childhood and cognitive assessment was done at the ages 8.5 and 11.5. The study reveals that children who were breast fed longer scored higher. Following their findings, Adair and Melissa (2005) concludes that breastfeeding is very important for cognitive development and should be encouraged even after the introduction of complementary foods.

A similar study was done by Anderson (1999) who examined the impact of duration of breastfeeding on cognitive development of Scandinavian children. Dealing with a population of 345 children, the three recorded data on breastfeeding during the first year of life. The study was followed for a period of the first five years of life. An evaluation of neuromotor development was carried out at the ages of 1 and 5 years respectively. Findings from their study reveal that a longer breast feeding duration benefits cognitive development. However, they recognized the fact that other factors like maternal intelligence, age, and education can also affect the cognitive development of children. Even after incorporating these in their study, the adjusted results still show the same pattern. Children breast fed for a period of 3 months scored poorer than those breast fed for at least six months. The study however did not find any clear link between breastfeeding and cognitive development at thirteen months or five years thus taking them back to the generalization that breastfeeding is very important especially during the first year of a child's life.

Breast Feeding and Cognitive Development

Literature on the importance of breast feeding on cognitive development is immense and the results are similar emphasizing the importance of breast milk. Despite the many supporting literature their findings are unconvincing to the opponents as the results are merely based on observational studies. Studies however have managed to dispute the fact that maternal socio-economic status also plays a role as some studies have statistically control for socio-economic differences. Some studies have even controlled statistically for maternal IQ with most results being slightly different but a significant effect of breast milk still show (Angelsen, 2001; Anderson1999). There is also the problem that these benefits could be confounded by differences in mother's behavior and interaction with the infant which equally play a significant psychological role in cognitive development. Such differences are very difficult to control in any observational study leave alone measuring them thus posing a methodological problem.

No matter the methodological problems associated with research studies based on this topic, the available literature has managed to prove its rationale. As a nurse, this is a very important topic that should be incorporated in antenatal and post natal programs. Nurses should be able to teach expectant mothers on the importance of breast feeding not only as an immunity booster but also for cognitive development. I have personally been inspired by the available literature on this topic and strongly believe fellow nurses should do something especially at this time that infant formula feeds are slowly replacing breast milk.

Best practices based on evidence scientist

Best practice is an essential tool for nurses especially those who are committed to excellence. But what does this jargon stand for? Best practice refers to a collection of clinical procedures, interventions and treatments that are geared towards achieving best possible results both to the patient and the concerned heath care facility (Lippincott and Wilkins, 2006). This is always arrived at through a study of available literature to find recommendations as well as collection of public views.

Based on the literature reviewed on this topic, it is clear that breast feeding play an important role in cognitive development. This evidence is good enough to campaign for exclusive breast feeding for at least six months and should even be continued after weaning.

Health care professionals should provide parents with the necessary information regarding the important role played by breast feeding in brain development to help them make informed decisions.

In cases where direct breast feeding is impossible as in HIV positive mothers, human milk should be provided as an alternative. This can only be made possible through intensive breast feeding campaigns (Rogan and Gladen 1993).

Contrary to the well documented importance of breast feeding for cognitive development, most mothers are currently shying away from this very important practice. With infant formula readily available in the market, mothers are increasingly moving away from the traditional norm of exclusive breast feeding. Besides mothers are currently involved in paid employments thus have very little time for their babies hence artificial feeds are increasingly becoming an option.

To this end I strongly recommend that breast feeding should never be supplemented for at whatever cost. Mothers should be encouraged to exclusively breast feed their babies at leased for the first six months. Incentives can be introduced to lure women towards this act. Furthermore, health care workers should be equally trained on the importance of breast feeding for cognitive development. Since this group work directly at the community level, it will be easier to use them to disseminate such important information. Besides, health care workers are basically members of the same community they operate in, so it will be much easier for them to be understood.

Women who are on paid employment should be encouraged to pump and use other options like bottle feeding so long as the milk is their own. Employers can also be encouraged to come up with baby nursery centre within to ensure infants are kept close to their mothers and can easily be breastfed during break hours (Rogan and Gladen 1993). Extension of the current maternity leave period is equally very important to ensure that mothers spend longer time with their children before resuming duties.

Suggestions for future research and their feasibility for best practice

From the literature reviewed, it was clear that all the previous examinations performed on this topic were merely observational studies. More comprehensive research needs to be done to clarify exactly how breast milk influences neurodevelopment. There is need for clinical studies to elucidate this. A comparative study using other important foods associated with neurodevelopment should be considered. In simple terms, an evaluation of the nutrient components of breast milk should be done to assert it's much talked of advantage. This can form a good research basis for medical practitioners. Only through such interventions, a clear distinct will be established.

Besides, all the studies done on this topic were conducted in developed countries despite the issue of socio-economic status as a confounding factor. I therefore suggest more studies in the least developed countries to establish whether the results still give breast milk an advantage over artificial foods. If the results come out the same, then it will be easier for health care professionals in those countries to promote breast feeding.

Finally I suggest that future studies should also incorporate the role played by maternal nutrient intake during the period of breast feeding. One cannot underestimate this since it is clear that the food a mother consume directly affects the nutritional value of her milk and of course the subsequent nutrient intake by the child. Probably mothers who feed on protein rich food like fish could bring up infants with a better developed brain. Such a study if proved right can really form good basis for advice to mothers on the type of food to eat during the gestation period and thus better developed cognitive function of their children.

More research on the duration of breast feeding should also be carried out. The current practice recommends exclusive breast feeding for a period of six months after birth. From what I noticed in the literature reviewed, some studies encouraged breast feeding beyond one year while others state it has no significance after nine months. A clear investigative study should be carried out to examine these accusations. This can also help health care professionals in advising mothers on exactly how long they should breast feed their babies.

Conclusion

Breast feeding is such an important practice not only for infants' immune system but cognitive development as well. Although many confounding factors exist studies have succeeded in asserting the fact that breast feeding directly contributes to high IQ, better cognitive function and verbal capability. The duration of breast feeding is equally a very important contributing factor. It was clear from the literature reviewed that a short breast feeding period, 3 months, is associated with low results while any additional month of breast feeding of up to one year is associated with high results. The importance breast milk accord neuro-motor development is the same both for children born pre-term and those born in term. To this end I still advocate for the promotion of breast feeding. Nurses as well as pediatrics should give mothers the necessary information to help the make informed decisions. I also recommend more research on this topic especially those geared towards medical studies as opposed to observational studies.

References

_____ (2004): *Breast Feeding Best practice Guidelines:* Retrieved 29th October 2010 from: http://www.pdfchaser.com/BREASTFE-ED-ING-Best-Practice-Guidelines.html

Adair, L & Daniels, M (2005) Breast feeding Influences Cognitive Development in Filipino: *Journal of Nutrition American Society for Nutrition* 135: 2589-2595.

Anderson, J (1999): Breastfeeding and Cognitive Development: a meta-analysis. American *Journal of Clinical Nutrition, Vol.70, No4, 525-535*

Angelsen N (2001): *Breast feeding and cognitive development at age 1 and 5 years. Archives of Disease in Children*; 85: 183-188. Retrieved 29th October 2010 from http://adc.bmj.com/content/85/3/183

Hoefer C & Hardy M (1929): Later Development of Breast Fed and Artificially Fed Infants. *JAMA, 92: 615-9*

Lippincott W & Wilkins, S (2006): *Best practice: evidence-based nursing procedures*: 2 edn. USA: Judith A Schilling McCann

Lucas A M (1992): *Breast Milk and Subsequent Intelligence Quotient in Children Born Pre-Term.* Lancet, 339(8788): 261-264

Morley, R & Lucas, A (2010): *Nutrition and Cognitive development. London*: Institute of Child Health. Retrieved 29th October 2010 from: http://bmb.oxfordjournals.org/content/53/1/123.full.pdf

Rogan W, & Gladen B (1993): *Breast feeding and Cognitive Development*: Early Human Development. 31:181-93